Nurse Report Notebook

MW00890284

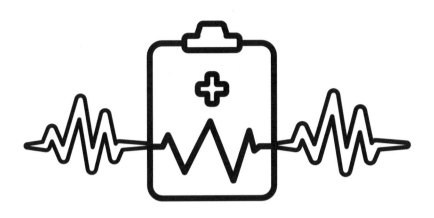

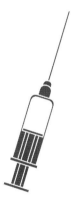

THIS BOOK BELONGS TO:

_____

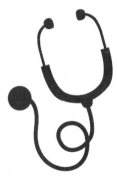

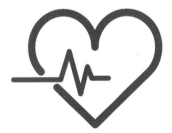

Simply Divine Journals

🩺 Nurse Report Sheet 〜♡

Name:

Code:

Room #:

Allergies:

Isolation:

DX:

PMH:

Neuro:

CV

Resp:

GI/GU:

Skin:

IV'S/Gtt:

Labs:

Notes/Plan:

- _____
- _____
- _____
- _____
- _____

Nurse Report Sheet

Name:

Code:

Room #:

Allergies:

Isolation:

DX:

PMH:

Neuro:

CV

Resp:

GI/GU:

Skin:

IV'S/Gtt:

Labs:

Notes/Plan:

- _____
- _____
- _____
- _____
- _____

Nurse Report Sheet

Name:

Code:

Room #:

Allergies:

Isolation:

DX:

PMH:

Neuro:

CV

Resp:

GI/GU:

Skin:

IV'S/Gtt:

Labs:

Notes/Plan:

- _____
- _____
- _____
- _____
- _____

Nurse Report Sheet

Name:

Code:

Room #:

Allergies:

Isolation:

DX:

PMH:

Neuro:

CV

Resp:

GI/GU:

Skin:

IV'S/Gtt:

Labs:

Notes/Plan:

- _____
- _____
- _____
- _____
- _____

Nurse Report Sheet

Name:

Code:

Room #:

Allergies:

Isolation:

DX:

PMH:

Neuro:

CV

Resp:

GI/GU:

Skin:

IV'S/Gtt:

Labs:

Notes/Plan:

- _____
- _____
- _____
- _____
- _____

Nurse Report Sheet

Name:

Code:

Room #:

Allergies:

Isolation:

DX:

PMH:

Neuro:

CV

Resp:

GI/GU:

Skin:

IV'S/Gtt:

Labs:

Notes/Plan:

- _____
- _____
- _____
- _____
- _____

🩺 Nurse Report Sheet 〰♡

Name:

Code:

Room #:

Allergies:

Isolation:

DX:

PMH:

Neuro:

CV

Resp:

GI/GU:

Skin:

IV'S/Gtt:

Labs:

Notes/Plan:

- _____
- _____
- _____
- _____
- _____

Nurse Report Sheet

Name:	Code:	Room #:

Allergies:	Isolation:

DX:

PMH:

Neuro:	CV

Resp:	GI/GU:

Skin:	IV'S/Gtt:

Labs:

Notes/Plan:
- _____
- _____
- _____
- _____
- _____

Nurse Report Sheet

Name:

Code:

Room #:

Allergies:

Isolation:

DX:

PMH:

Neuro:

CV

Resp:

GI/GU:

Skin:

IV'S/Gtt:

Labs:

Notes/Plan:

- _____
- _____
- _____
- _____
- _____

Nurse Report Sheet

Name:

Code:

Room #:

Allergies:

Isolation:

DX:

PMH:

Neuro:

CV

Resp:

GI/GU:

Skin:

IV'S/Gtt:

Labs:

Notes/Plan:
- _____
- _____
- _____
- _____
- _____

🩺 Nurse Report Sheet ∿♡

Name:

Code:

Room #:

Allergies:

Isolation:

DX:

PMH:

Neuro:

CV

Resp:

GI/GU:

Skin:

IV'S/Gtt:

Labs:

Notes/Plan:

- _____
- _____
- _____
- _____
- _____

Nurse Report Sheet

Name:

Code:

Room #:

Allergies:

Isolation:

DX:

PMH:

Neuro:

CV

Resp:

GI/GU:

Skin:

IV'S/Gtt:

Labs:

Notes/Plan:

- _____
- _____
- _____
- _____
- _____

🏥 Nurse Report Sheet ⎍♡

| Name: | Code: | Room #: |

| Allergies: | Isolation: |

DX:

PMH:

Neuro:	CV

Resp:	GI/GU:

Skin:	IV'S/Gtt:

Labs:	Notes/Plan: • _____ • _____ • _____ • _____ • _____

Nurse Report Sheet

Name:

Code:

Room #:

Allergies:

Isolation:

DX:

PMH:

Neuro:

CV

Resp:

GI/GU:

Skin:

IV'S/Gtt:

Labs:

Notes/Plan:

- _____
- _____
- _____
- _____
- _____

Nurse Report Sheet

Name:

Code:

Room #:

Allergies:

Isolation:

DX:

PMH:

Neuro:

CV

Resp:

GI/GU:

Skin:

IV'S/Gtt:

Labs:

Notes/Plan:

- _____
- _____
- _____
- _____
- _____

Nurse Report Sheet

Name:

Code:

Room #:

Allergies:

Isolation:

DX:

PMH:

Neuro:

CV

Resp:

GI/GU:

Skin:

IV'S/Gtt:

Labs:

Notes/Plan:
- _____
- _____
- _____
- _____
- _____

Nurse Report Sheet

Name:

Code:

Room #:

Allergies:

Isolation:

DX:

PMH:

Neuro:

CV

Resp:

GI/GU:

Skin:

IV'S/Gtt:

Labs:

Notes/Plan:

- _____
- _____
- _____
- _____
- _____

Nurse Report Sheet

Name:

Code:

Room #:

Allergies:

Isolation:

DX:

PMH:

Neuro:

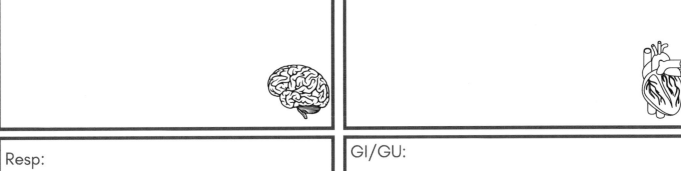

CV

Resp:

GI/GU:

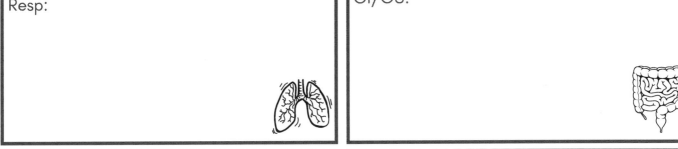

Skin:

IV'S/Gtt:

Labs:

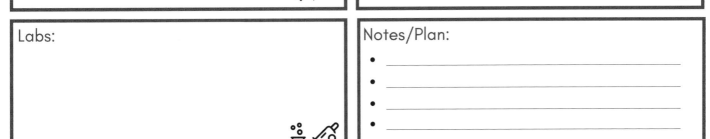

Notes/Plan:

- _____
- _____
- _____
- _____
- _____

Nurse Report Sheet

Name:

Code:

Room #:

Allergies:

Isolation:

DX:

PMH:

Neuro:

CV

Resp:

GI/GU:

Skin:

IV'S/Gtt:

Labs:

Notes/Plan:

- _____
- _____
- _____
- _____
- _____

Nurse Report Sheet

Name:

Code:

Room #:

Allergies:

Isolation:

DX:

PMH:

Neuro:

CV

Resp:

GI/GU:

Skin:

IV'S/Gtt:

Labs:

Notes/Plan:

- _____
- _____
- _____
- _____
- _____

Nurse Report Sheet

Name:

Code:

Room #:

Allergies:

Isolation:

DX:

PMH:

Neuro:

CV

Resp:

GI/GU:

Skin:

IV'S/Gtt:

Labs:

Notes/Plan:

- _____
- _____
- _____
- _____
- _____

Nurse Report Sheet

Name:

Code:

Room #:

Allergies:

Isolation:

DX:

PMH:

Neuro:

CV

Resp:

GI/GU:

Skin:

IV'S/Gtt:

Labs:

Notes/Plan:

- _____
- _____
- _____
- _____
- _____

🧑‍⚕️ Nurse Report Sheet 〜♡

Name: **Code:**   **Room #:**

Allergies: **Isolation:**

DX:

PMH:

Neuro: **CV**

Resp: **GI/GU:**

Skin: **IV'S/Gtt:**

Labs: **Notes/Plan:**

- _____
- _____
- _____
- _____
- _____

Nurse Report Sheet

Name:

Code:

Room #:

Allergies:

Isolation:

DX:

PMH:

Neuro:

CV

Resp:

GI/GU:

Skin:

IV'S/Gtt:

Labs:

Notes/Plan:

- _____
- _____
- _____
- _____
- _____

🩺 Nurse Report Sheet 〰️♡

Name:

Code:

Room #:

Allergies:

Isolation:

DX:

PMH:

Neuro:

CV

Resp:

GI/GU:

Skin:

IV'S/Gtt:

Labs:

Notes/Plan:
- _____
- _____
- _____
- _____
- _____

Nurse Report Sheet

Name:

Code:

Room #:

Allergies:

Isolation:

DX:

PMH:

Neuro:

CV

Resp:

GI/GU:

Skin:

IV'S/Gtt:

Labs:

Notes/Plan:

- _____
- _____
- _____
- _____
- _____

🩺 Nurse Report Sheet ⏤♡

Name:

Code:

Room #:

Allergies:

Isolation:

DX:

PMH:

Neuro:

CV

Resp:

GI/GU:

Skin:

IV'S/Gtt:

Labs:

Notes/Plan:

- _____
- _____
- _____
- _____
- _____

Nurse Report Sheet

Name:

Code:

Room #:

Allergies:

Isolation:

DX:

PMH:

Neuro:

CV

Resp:

GI/GU:

Skin:

IV'S/Gtt:

Labs:

Notes/Plan:
- _____
- _____
- _____
- _____
- _____

Nurse Report Sheet

Name:	Code:	Room #:

Allergies:	Isolation:

DX:

PMH:

Neuro:	CV

Resp:	GI/GU:

Skin:	IV'S/Gtt:

Labs:	Notes/Plan:
	• _____
	• _____
	• _____
	• _____
	• _____

Nurse Report Sheet

Name:

Code:

Room #:

Allergies:

Isolation:

DX:

PMH:

Neuro:

CV

Resp:

GI/GU:

Skin:

IV'S/Gtt:

Labs:

Notes/Plan:

- _____
- _____
- _____
- _____
- _____

🩺 Nurse Report Sheet 〰️♡

Name: **Code:**   **Room #:**

Allergies: **Isolation:**

DX:

PMH:

Neuro: **CV**

Resp: **GI/GU:**

Skin: **IV'S/Gtt:**

Labs: **Notes/Plan:**

- _____
- _____
- _____
- _____
- _____

Nurse Report Sheet

Name:

Code:

Room #:

Allergies:

Isolation:

DX:

PMH:

Neuro:

CV

Resp:

GI/GU:

Skin:

IV'S/Gtt:

Labs:

Notes/Plan:

- _____
- _____
- _____
- _____
- _____

Nurse Report Sheet

Name:	Code:	Room #:

Allergies:	Isolation:

DX:

PMH:

Neuro:	CV

Resp:	GI/GU:

Skin:	IV'S/Gtt:

Labs:

Notes/Plan:
- _____
- _____
- _____
- _____
- _____

🏥 Nurse Report Sheet 〰️♡

Name:

Code:

Room #:

Allergies:

Isolation:

DX:

PMH:

Neuro:

CV

Resp:

GI/GU:

Skin:

IV'S/Gtt:

Labs:

Notes/Plan:

- _____
- _____
- _____
- _____
- _____

Nurse Report Sheet

Name:

Code:

Room #:

Allergies:

Isolation:

DX:

PMH:

Neuro:

CV

Resp:

GI/GU:

Skin:

IV'S/Gtt:

Labs:

Notes/Plan:

- _____
- _____
- _____
- _____
- _____

Nurse Report Sheet

Name:

Code:

Room #:

Allergies:

Isolation:

DX:

PMH:

Neuro:

CV

Resp:

GI/GU:

Skin:

IV'S/Gtt:

Labs:

Notes/Plan:
- _____
- _____
- _____
- _____
- _____

Nurse Report Sheet

Name:

Code:

Room #:

Allergies:

Isolation:

DX:

PMH:

Neuro:

CV

Resp:

GI/GU:

Skin:

IV'S/Gtt:

Labs:

Notes/Plan:
- _____
- _____
- _____
- _____
- _____

Nurse Report Sheet

Name:	Code:	Room #:

Allergies:

Isolation:

DX:

PMH:

Neuro:

CV

Resp:

GI/GU:

Skin:

IV'S/Gtt:

Labs:

Notes/Plan:

- _____
- _____
- _____
- _____
- _____

👲 Nurse Report Sheet 〰️♡

Name:	Code:	Room #:

Allergies:	Isolation:

DX:

PMH:

Neuro:

CV

Resp:

GI/GU:

Skin:

IV'S/Gtt:

Labs:

Notes/Plan:

- _____
- _____
- _____
- _____
- _____

Nurse Report Sheet

Name:

Code:

Room #:

Allergies:

Isolation:

DX:

PMH:

Neuro:

CV

Resp:

GI/GU:

Skin:

IV'S/Gtt:

Labs:

Notes/Plan:

- _____
- _____
- _____
- _____
- _____

Nurse Report Sheet

Name:

Code:

Room #:

Allergies:

Isolation:

DX:

PMH:

Neuro:

CV

Resp:

GI/GU:

Skin:

IV'S/Gtt:

Labs:

Notes/Plan:

- _____
- _____
- _____
- _____
- _____

Nurse Report Sheet

Name:

Code:

Room #:

Allergies:

Isolation:

DX:

PMH:

Neuro:

CV

Resp:

GI/GU:

Skin:

IV'S/Gtt:

Labs:

Notes/Plan:
- _____
- _____
- _____
- _____
- _____

Nurse Report Sheet

Name:

Code:

Room #:

Allergies:

Isolation:

DX:

PMH:

Neuro:

CV

Resp:

GI/GU:

Skin:

IV'S/Gtt:

Labs:

Notes/Plan:

- _____
- _____
- _____
- _____
- _____

Nurse Report Sheet

Name:

Code:

Room #:

Allergies:

Isolation:

DX:

PMH:

Neuro:

CV

Resp:

GI/GU:

Skin:

IV'S/Gtt:

Labs:

Notes/Plan:

- _____
- _____
- _____
- _____
- _____

Nurse Report Sheet

Name:

Code:

Room #:

Allergies:

Isolation:

DX:

PMH:

Neuro:

CV

Resp:

GI/GU:

Skin:

IV'S/Gtt:

Labs:

Notes/Plan:
- _____
- _____
- _____
- _____
- _____

Nurse Report Sheet

Name:

Code:

Room #:

Allergies:

Isolation:

DX:

PMH:

Neuro:

CV

Resp:

GI/GU:

Skin:

IV'S/Gtt:

Labs:

Notes/Plan:
- _____
- _____
- _____
- _____
- _____

Nurse Report Sheet

Name:

Code:

Room #:

Allergies:

Isolation:

DX:

PMH:

Neuro:

CV

Resp:

GI/GU:

Skin:

IV'S/Gtt:

Labs:

Notes/Plan:

- _____
- _____
- _____
- _____
- _____

Nurse Report Sheet

| Name: | Code: | Room #: |

| Allergies: | Isolation: |

DX:

PMH:

Neuro:

CV

Resp:

GI/GU:

Skin:

IV'S/Gtt:

Labs:

Notes/Plan:
- _____
- _____
- _____
- _____
- _____

Nurse Report Sheet

Name:

Code:

Room #:

Allergies:

Isolation:

DX:

PMH:

Neuro:

CV

Resp:

GI/GU:

Skin:

IV'S/Gtt:

Labs:

Notes/Plan:
- _____
- _____
- _____
- _____
- _____

Nurse Report Sheet

Name:

Code:

Room #:

Allergies:

Isolation:

DX:

PMH:

Neuro:

CV

Resp:

GI/GU:

Skin:

IV'S/Gtt:

Labs:

Notes/Plan:

- _____
- _____
- _____
- _____
- _____

🪺 Nurse Report Sheet ⩗♡

Name:

Code:

Room #:

Allergies:

Isolation:

DX:

PMH:

Neuro:

CV

Resp:

GI/GU:

Skin:

IV'S/Gtt:

Labs:

Notes/Plan:

- _____
- _____
- _____
- _____
- _____

Nurse Report Sheet

Name:

Code:

Room #:

Allergies:

Isolation:

DX:

PMH:

Neuro:

CV

Resp:

GI/GU:

Skin:

IV'S/Gtt:

Labs:

Notes/Plan:

- _____
- _____
- _____
- _____
- _____

Nurse Report Sheet

Name:

Code:

Room #:

Allergies:

Isolation:

DX:

PMH:

Neuro:

CV

Resp:

GI/GU:

Skin:

IV'S/Gtt:

Labs:

Notes/Plan:
- _____
- _____
- _____
- _____
- _____

Nurse Report Sheet

Name:

Code:

Room #:

Allergies:

Isolation:

DX:

PMH:

Neuro:

CV

Resp:

GI/GU:

Skin:

IV'S/Gtt:

Labs:

Notes/Plan:
- _____
- _____
- _____
- _____
- _____

🧑‍⚕️ Nurse Report Sheet ∿♡

| Name: | Code: | Room #: |

Allergies:

Isolation:

DX:

PMH:

Neuro:

CV

Resp:

GI/GU:

Skin:

IV'S/Gtt:

Labs:

Notes/Plan:
- _____
- _____
- _____
- _____
- _____

Nurse Report Sheet

Name:

Code:

Room #:

Allergies:

Isolation:

DX:

PMH:

Neuro:

CV

Resp:

GI/GU:

Skin:

IV'S/Gtt:

Labs:

Notes/Plan:
- _____
- _____
- _____
- _____
- _____

Nurse Report Sheet

Name:

Code:

Room #:

Allergies:

Isolation:

DX:

PMH:

Neuro:

CV

Resp:

GI/GU:

Skin:

IV'S/Gtt:

Labs:

Notes/Plan:

- _____
- _____
- _____
- _____
- _____

Nurse Report Sheet

Name:

Code:

Room #:

Allergies:

Isolation:

DX:

PMH:

Neuro:

CV

Resp:

GI/GU:

Skin:

IV'S/Gtt:

Labs:

Notes/Plan:
- _____
- _____
- _____
- _____
- _____

Nurse Report Sheet

Name:

Code:

Room #:

Allergies:

Isolation:

DX:

PMH:

Neuro:

CV

Resp:

GI/GU:

Skin:

IV'S/Gtt:

Labs:

Notes/Plan:

- _____
- _____
- _____
- _____
- _____

Nurse Report Sheet

Name:

Code:

Room #:

Allergies:

Isolation:

DX:

PMH:

Neuro:

CV

Resp:

GI/GU:

Skin:

IV'S/Gtt:

Labs:

Notes/Plan:

- _____
- _____
- _____
- _____
- _____

Nurse Report Sheet

Name:	Code:	Room #:

Allergies:	Isolation:

DX:

PMH:

Neuro:

CV

Resp:

GI/GU:

Skin:

IV'S/Gtt:

Labs:

Notes/Plan:
- _____
- _____
- _____
- _____
- _____

Nurse Report Sheet

Name:

Code:

Room #:

Allergies:

Isolation:

DX:

PMH:

Neuro:

CV

Resp:

GI/GU:

Skin:

IV'S/Gtt:

Labs:

Notes/Plan:

- _____
- _____
- _____
- _____
- _____

Nurse Report Sheet

Name:

Code:

Room #:

Allergies:

Isolation:

DX:

PMH:

Neuro:

CV

Resp:

GI/GU:

Skin:

IV'S/Gtt:

Labs:

Notes/Plan:
- _____
- _____
- _____
- _____
- _____

Nurse Report Sheet

Name:	Code:	Room #:

Allergies:	Isolation:

DX:

PMH:

Neuro:

CV

Resp:

GI/GU:

Skin:

IV'S/Gtt:

Labs:

Notes/Plan:
- _____
- _____
- _____
- _____
- _____

Nurse Report Sheet

Name:	Code:	Room #:

Allergies:	Isolation:

DX:

PMH:

Neuro:

CV

Resp:

GI/GU:

Skin:

IV'S/Gtt:

Labs:

Notes/Plan:
- _____
- _____
- _____
- _____
- _____

Nurse Report Sheet

Name:

Code:

Room #:

Allergies:

Isolation:

DX:

PMH:

Neuro:

CV

Resp:

GI/GU:

Skin:

IV'S/Gtt:

Labs:

Notes/Plan:

- _____
- _____
- _____
- _____
- _____

Nurse Report Sheet

Name:

Code:

Room #:

Allergies:

Isolation:

DX:

PMH:

Neuro:

CV

Resp:

GI/GU:

Skin:

IV'S/Gtt:

Labs:

Notes/Plan:

- _____
- _____
- _____
- _____
- _____

Nurse Report Sheet

Name:

Code:

Room #:

Allergies:

Isolation:

DX:

PMH:

Neuro:

CV

Resp:

GI/GU:

Skin:

IV'S/Gtt:

Labs:

Notes/Plan:
- _____
- _____
- _____
- _____
- _____

Nurse Report Sheet

Name:	Code:	Room #:

Allergies:	Isolation:

DX:

PMH:

Neuro:

CV

Resp:

GI/GU:

Skin:

IV'S/Gtt:

Labs:

Notes/Plan:
- _____
- _____
- _____
- _____
- _____

Nurse Report Sheet

Name:

Code:

Room #:

Allergies:

Isolation:

DX:

PMH:

Neuro:

CV

Resp:

GI/GU:

Skin:

IV'S/Gtt:

Labs:

Notes/Plan:

- _____
- _____
- _____
- _____
- _____

Nurse Report Sheet

Name:	Code:	Room #:

Allergies:	Isolation:

DX:

PMH:

Neuro:

CV

Resp:

GI/GU:

Skin:

IV'S/Gtt:

Labs:

Notes/Plan:
- _____
- _____
- _____
- _____
- _____

Nurse Report Sheet

Name:

Code:

Room #:

Allergies:

Isolation:

DX:

PMH:

Neuro:

CV

Resp:

GI/GU:

Skin:

IV'S/Gtt:

Labs:

Notes/Plan:

- _____
- _____
- _____
- _____
- _____

🩺 Nurse Report Sheet 〜♡

Name:

Code:

Room #:

Allergies:

Isolation:

DX:

PMH:

Neuro:

CV

Resp:

GI/GU:

Skin:

IV'S/Gtt:

Labs:

Notes/Plan:
- _____
- _____
- _____
- _____
- _____

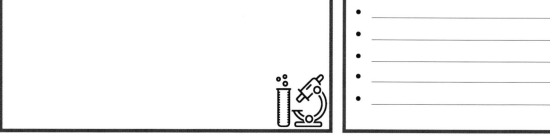

Nurse Report Sheet

Name:

Code:

Room #:

Allergies:

Isolation:

DX:

PMH:

Neuro:

CV

Resp:

GI/GU:

Skin:

IV'S/Gtt:

Labs:

Notes/Plan:

- _____
- _____
- _____
- _____
- _____

🏥 Nurse Report Sheet 〰️♡

Name:

Code:

Room #:

Allergies:

Isolation:

DX:

PMH:

Neuro:

CV

Resp:

GI/GU:

Skin:

IV'S/Gtt:

Labs:

Notes/Plan:

- _____
- _____
- _____
- _____
- _____

Nurse Report Sheet

Name:

Code:

Room #:

Allergies:

Isolation:

DX:

PMH:

Neuro:

CV

Resp:

GI/GU:

Skin:

IV'S/Gtt:

Labs:

Notes/Plan:

- _____
- _____
- _____
- _____
- _____

Nurse Report Sheet

Name:

Code:

Room #:

Allergies:

Isolation:

DX:

PMH:

Neuro:

CV

Resp:

GI/GU:

Skin:

IV'S/Gtt:

Labs:

Notes/Plan:

- _____
- _____
- _____
- _____
- _____

Nurse Report Sheet

Name:

Code:

Room #:

Allergies:

Isolation:

DX:

PMH:

Neuro:

CV

Resp:

GI/GU:

Skin:

IV'S/Gtt:

Labs:

Notes/Plan:
- _____
- _____
- _____
- _____
- _____

Nurse Report Sheet

Name:

Code:

Room #:

Allergies:

Isolation:

DX:

PMH:

Neuro:

CV

Resp:

GI/GU:

Skin:

IV'S/Gtt:

Labs:

Notes/Plan:

- _____
- _____
- _____
- _____
- _____

Nurse Report Sheet

Name:	Code:	Room #:

Allergies:

Isolation:

DX:

PMH:

Neuro:

CV

Resp:

GI/GU:

Skin:

IV'S/Gtt:

Labs:

Notes/Plan:
- _____
- _____
- _____
- _____
- _____

Nurse Report Sheet

Name:

Code:

Room #:

Allergies:

Isolation:

DX:

PMH:

Neuro:

CV

Resp:

GI/GU:

Skin:

IV'S/Gtt:

Labs:

Notes/Plan:

- _____
- _____
- _____
- _____
- _____

Nurse Report Sheet

Name:

Code:

Room #:

Allergies:

Isolation:

DX:

PMH:

Neuro:

CV

Resp:

GI/GU:

Skin:

IV'S/Gtt:

Labs:

Notes/Plan:

- _____
- _____
- _____
- _____
- _____

Nurse Report Sheet

Name:

Code:

Room #:

Allergies:

Isolation:

DX:

PMH:

Neuro:

CV

Resp:

GI/GU:

Skin:

IV'S/Gtt:

Labs:

Notes/Plan:

- _____
- _____
- _____
- _____
- _____

Nurse Report Sheet

Name:

Code:

Room #:

Allergies:

Isolation:

DX:

PMH:

Neuro:

CV

Resp:

GI/GU:

Skin:

IV'S/Gtt:

Labs:

Notes/Plan:

- _____
- _____
- _____
- _____
- _____

Nurse Report Sheet

Name:	Code:	Room #:

Allergies:	Isolation:

DX:

PMH:

Neuro:	CV

Resp:	GI/GU:

Skin:	IV'S/Gtt:

Labs:	Notes/Plan: • _____ • _____ • _____ • _____ • _____

Nurse Report Sheet

Name:

Code:

Room #:

Allergies:

Isolation:

DX:

PMH:

Neuro:

CV

Resp:

GI/GU:

Skin:

IV'S/Gtt:

Labs:

Notes/Plan:
- _____
- _____
- _____
- _____
- _____

Nurse Report Sheet

Name:

Code:

Room #:

Allergies:

Isolation:

DX:

PMH:

Neuro:

CV

Resp:

GI/GU:

Skin:

IV'S/Gtt:

Labs:

Notes/Plan:

- _____
- _____
- _____
- _____
- _____

Nurse Report Sheet

Name:	Code:	Room #:

Allergies:	Isolation:

DX:

PMH:

Neuro:

CV

Resp:

GI/GU:

Skin:

IV'S/Gtt:

Labs:

Notes/Plan:

- _____
- _____
- _____
- _____
- _____

Nurse Report Sheet

Name:	Code:	Room #:

Allergies:	Isolation:

DX:

PMH:

Neuro:	CV

Resp:	GI/GU:

Skin:	IV'S/Gtt:

Labs:

Notes/Plan:
- _____
- _____
- _____
- _____
- _____

Nurse Report Sheet

Name:

Code:

Room #:

Allergies:

Isolation:

DX:

PMH:

Neuro:

CV

Resp:

GI/GU:

Skin:

IV'S/Gtt:

Labs:

Notes/Plan:

- _____
- _____
- _____
- _____
- _____

Nurse Report Sheet

Name:

Code:

Room #:

Allergies:

Isolation:

DX:

PMH:

Neuro:

CV

Resp:

GI/GU:

Skin:

IV'S/Gtt:

Labs:

Notes/Plan:

- _____
- _____
- _____
- _____
- _____

Nurse Report Sheet

Name:

Code:

Room #:

Allergies:

Isolation:

DX:

PMH:

Neuro:

CV

Resp:

GI/GU:

Skin:

IV'S/Gtt:

Labs:

Notes/Plan:
- _____
- _____
- _____
- _____
- _____

Nurse Report Sheet

Name:	Code:	Room #:

Allergies:

Isolation:

DX:

PMH:

Neuro:	CV

Resp:	GI/GU:

Skin:	IV'S/Gtt:

Labs:

Notes/Plan:
- _____
- _____
- _____
- _____
- _____

Nurse Report Sheet

Name:

Code:

Room #:

Allergies:

Isolation:

DX:

PMH:

Neuro:

CV

Resp:

GI/GU:

Skin:

IV'S/Gtt:

Labs:

Notes/Plan:

- _____
- _____
- _____
- _____
- _____

Nurse Report Sheet

Name:	Code:	Room #:

Allergies:	Isolation:

DX:

PMH:

Neuro:	CV

Resp:	GI/GU:

Skin:	IV'S/Gtt:

Labs:	Notes/Plan:
	• _____
	• _____
	• _____
	• _____
	• _____

Nurse Report Sheet

Name:

Code:

Room #:

Allergies:

Isolation:

DX:

PMH:

Neuro:

CV

Resp:

GI/GU:

Skin:

IV'S/Gtt:

Labs:

Notes/Plan:
- _____
- _____
- _____
- _____
- _____

Nurse Report Sheet

Name:	Code:	Room #:

Allergies:	Isolation:

DX:

PMH:

Neuro:

CV

Resp:

GI/GU:

Skin:

IV'S/Gtt:

Labs:

Notes/Plan:
- _____
- _____
- _____
- _____
- _____

Nurse Report Sheet

Name:

Code:

Room #:

Allergies:

Isolation:

DX:

PMH:

Neuro:

CV

Resp:

GI/GU:

Skin:

IV'S/Gtt:

Labs:

Notes/Plan:

- _____
- _____
- _____
- _____
- _____

Nurse Report Sheet

Name:

Code:

Room #:

Allergies:

Isolation:

DX:

PMH:

Neuro:

CV

Resp:

GI/GU:

Skin:

IV'S/Gtt:

Labs:

Notes/Plan:

- _____
- _____
- _____
- _____
- _____

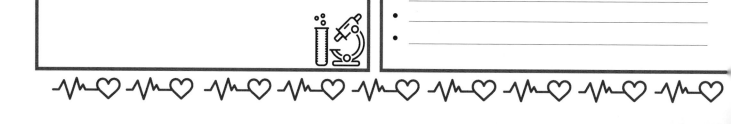

Nurse Report Sheet

Name:

Code:

Room #:

Allergies:

Isolation:

DX:

PMH:

Neuro:

CV

Resp:

GI/GU:

Skin:

IV'S/Gtt:

Labs:

Notes/Plan:

- _____
- _____
- _____
- _____
- _____

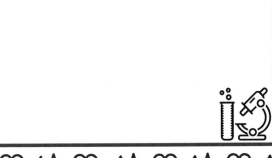

Nurse Report Sheet

Name:	Code:	Room #:

Allergies:	Isolation:

DX:

PMH:

Neuro:	CV

Resp:	GI/GU:

Skin:	IV'S/Gtt:

Labs:	Notes/Plan:
	• _____
	• _____
	• _____
	• _____
	• _____

Nurse Report Sheet

Name:

Code:

Room #:

Allergies:

Isolation:

DX:

PMH:

Neuro:

CV

Resp:

GI/GU:

Skin:

IV'S/Gtt:

Labs:

Notes/Plan:

- _____
- _____
- _____
- _____
- _____

Nurse Report Sheet

Name:

Code:

Room #:

Allergies:

Isolation:

DX:

PMH:

Neuro:

CV

Resp:

GI/GU:

Skin:

IV'S/Gtt:

Labs:

Notes/Plan:
- _____
- _____
- _____
- _____
- _____

Nurse Report Sheet

Name:

Code:

Room #:

Allergies:

Isolation:

DX:

PMH:

Neuro:

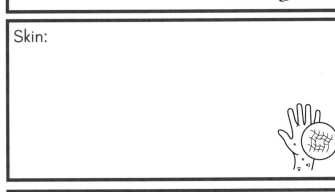

CV

Resp:

GI/GU:

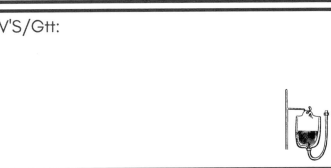

Skin:

IV'S/Gtt:

Labs:

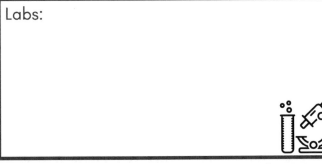

Notes/Plan:

- _____
- _____
- _____
- _____
- _____

Nurse Report Sheet

Name:

Code:

Room #:

Allergies:

Isolation:

DX:

PMH:

Neuro:

CV

Resp:

GI/GU:

Skin:

IV'S/Gtt:

Labs:

Notes/Plan:

- _____
- _____
- _____
- _____
- _____

Nurse Report Sheet

Name:	Code:	Room #:

Allergies:	Isolation:

DX:

PMH:

Neuro:	CV

Resp:	GI/GU:

Skin:	IV'S/Gtt:

Labs:

Notes/Plan:
- _____
- _____
- _____
- _____
- _____

Nurse Report Sheet

Name:	Code:	Room #:

Allergies:	Isolation:

DX:

PMH:

Neuro:	CV

Resp:	GI/GU:

Skin:	IV'S/Gtt:

Labs:	Notes/Plan:

Notes/Plan:
- _____
- _____
- _____
- _____
- _____

Nurse Report Sheet

Name:

Code:

Room #:

Allergies:

Isolation:

DX:

PMH:

Neuro:

CV

Resp:

GI/GU:

Skin:

IV'S/Gtt:

Labs:

Notes/Plan:

- _____
- _____
- _____
- _____
- _____

Nurse Report Sheet

Name:

Code:

Room #:

Allergies:

Isolation:

DX:

PMH:

Neuro:

CV

Resp:

GI/GU:

Skin:

IV'S/Gtt:

Labs:

Notes/Plan:
- _____
- _____
- _____
- _____
- _____

Nurse Report Sheet

Name:

Code:

Room #:

Allergies:

Isolation:

DX:

PMH:

Neuro:

CV

Resp:

GI/GU:

Skin:

IV'S/Gtt:

Labs:

Notes/Plan:

- _____
- _____
- _____
- _____
- _____

Nurse Report Sheet

Name:

Code:

Room #:

Allergies:

Isolation:

DX:

PMH:

Neuro:

CV

Resp:

GI/GU:

Skin:

IV'S/Gtt:

Labs:

Notes/Plan:

- _____
- _____
- _____
- _____
- _____

Nurse Report Sheet

Name:

Code:

Room #:

Allergies:

Isolation:

DX:

PMH:

Neuro:

CV

Resp:

GI/GU:

Skin:

IV'S/Gtt:

Labs:

Notes/Plan:

- _____
- _____
- _____
- _____
- _____

Nurse Report Sheet

Name:

Code:

Room #:

Allergies:

Isolation:

DX:

PMH:

Neuro:

CV

Resp:

GI/GU:

Skin:

IV'S/Gtt:

Labs:

Notes/Plan:
- _____
- _____
- _____
- _____
- _____

Nurse Report Sheet

Name:

Code:

Room #:

Allergies:

Isolation:

DX:

PMH:

Neuro:

CV

Resp:

GI/GU:

Skin:

IV'S/Gtt:

Labs:

Notes/Plan:

- _____
- _____
- _____
- _____
- _____

Nurse Report Sheet

Name:

Code:

Room #:

Allergies:

Isolation:

DX:

PMH:

Neuro:

CV

Resp:

GI/GU:

Skin:

IV'S/Gtt:

Labs:

Notes/Plan:

- _____
- _____
- _____
- _____
- _____

Nurse Report Sheet

Name:	Code:	Room #:

Allergies:	Isolation:

DX:

PMH:

Neuro:

CV

Resp:

GI/GU:

Skin:

IV'S/Gtt:

Labs:

Notes/Plan:

- _____
- _____
- _____
- _____
- _____

Nurse Report Sheet

Name:

Code:

Room #:

Allergies:

Isolation:

DX:

PMH:

Neuro:

CV

Resp:

GI/GU:

Skin:

IV'S/Gtt:

Labs:

Notes/Plan:
- _____
- _____
- _____
- _____
- _____

Nurse Report Sheet

Name:

Code:

Room #:

Allergies:

Isolation:

DX:

PMH:

Neuro:

CV

Resp:

GI/GU:

Skin:

IV'S/Gtt:

Labs:

Notes/Plan:

- _____
- _____
- _____
- _____
- _____

Nurse Report Sheet

Name:

Code:

Room #:

Allergies:

Isolation:

DX:

PMH:

Neuro:

CV

Resp:

GI/GU:

Skin:

IV'S/Gtt:

Labs:

Notes/Plan:
- _____
- _____
- _____
- _____
- _____

Nurse Report Sheet

Name:

Code:

Room #:

Allergies:

Isolation:

DX:

PMH:

Neuro:

CV

Resp:

GI/GU:

Skin:

IV'S/Gtt:

Labs:

Notes/Plan:

- _____
- _____
- _____
- _____
- _____

Nurse Report Sheet

Name:

Code:

Room #:

Allergies:

Isolation:

DX:

PMH:

Neuro:

CV

Resp:

GI/GU:

Skin:

IV'S/Gtt:

Labs:

Notes/Plan:

- _____
- _____
- _____
- _____
- _____

Nurse Report Sheet

Name:	Code:	Room #:

Allergies:	Isolation:

DX:

PMH:

Neuro:

CV

Resp:

GI/GU:

Skin:

IV'S/Gtt:

Labs:

Notes/Plan:

- _____
- _____
- _____
- _____
- _____

Nurse Report Sheet

Name:	Code:	Room #:

Allergies:	Isolation:

DX:

PMH:

Neuro:	CV

Resp:	GI/GU:

Skin:	IV'S/Gtt:

Labs:	Notes/Plan:

Notes/Plan:
- _____
- _____
- _____
- _____
- _____

Nurse Report Sheet

Name:

Code:

Room #:

Allergies:

Isolation:

DX:

PMH:

Neuro:

CV

Resp:

GI/GU:

Skin:

IV'S/Gtt:

Labs:

Notes/Plan:

- _____
- _____
- _____
- _____
- _____

Nurse Report Sheet

Name:

Code:

Room #:

Allergies:

Isolation:

DX:

PMH:

Neuro:

CV

Resp:

GI/GU:

Skin:

IV'S/Gtt:

Labs:

Notes/Plan:

- _____
- _____
- _____
- _____
- _____

Nurse Report Sheet

Name:

Code:

Room #:

Allergies:

Isolation:

DX:

PMH:

Neuro:

CV

Resp:

GI/GU:

Skin:

IV'S/Gtt:

Labs:

Notes/Plan:

- _____
- _____
- _____
- _____
- _____

Nurse Report Sheet

Name:	Code:	Room #:

Allergies:	Isolation:

DX:

PMH:

Neuro:	CV

Resp:	GI/GU:

Skin:	IV'S/Gtt:

Labs:

Notes/Plan:
- _____
- _____
- _____
- _____
- _____

Nurse Report Sheet

Name:

Code:

Room #:

Allergies:

Isolation:

DX:

PMH:

Neuro:

CV

Resp:

GI/GU:

Skin:

IV'S/Gtt:

Labs:

Notes/Plan:
- _____
- _____
- _____
- _____
- _____

Nurse Report Sheet

Name:

Code:

Room #:

Allergies:

Isolation:

DX:

PMH:

Neuro:

CV

Resp:

GI/GU:

Skin:

IV'S/Gtt:

Labs:

Notes/Plan:

- _____
- _____
- _____
- _____
- _____

Nurse Report Sheet

Name:

Code:

Room #:

Allergies:

Isolation:

DX:

PMH:

Neuro:

CV

Resp:

GI/GU:

Skin:

IV'S/Gtt:

Labs:

Notes/Plan:
- _____
- _____
- _____
- _____
- _____

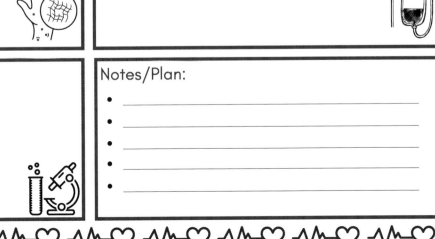

Nurse Report Sheet

Name:

Code:

Room #:

Allergies:

Isolation:

DX:

PMH:

Neuro:

CV

Resp:

GI/GU:

Skin:

IV'S/Gtt:

Labs:

Notes/Plan:
- _____
- _____
- _____
- _____
- _____

Nurse Report Sheet

Name:

Code:

Room #:

Allergies:

Isolation:

DX:

PMH:

Neuro:

CV

Resp:

GI/GU:

Skin:

IV'S/Gtt:

Labs:

Notes/Plan:

- _____
- _____
- _____
- _____
- _____

Nurse Report Sheet

Name:

Code:

Room #:

Allergies:

Isolation:

DX:

PMH:

Neuro:

CV

Resp:

GI/GU:

Skin:

IV'S/Gtt:

Labs:

Notes/Plan:

- _____
- _____
- _____
- _____
- _____

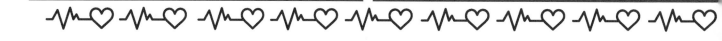

Nurse Report Sheet

Name:

Code:

Room #:

Allergies:

Isolation:

DX:

PMH:

Neuro:

CV

Resp:

GI/GU:

Skin:

IV'S/Gtt:

Labs:

Notes/Plan:
- _____
- _____
- _____
- _____
- _____

Nurse Report Sheet

| Name: | Code: | Room #: |

| Allergies: | Isolation: |

DX:

PMH:

| Neuro: | CV |

| Resp: | GI/GU: |

| Skin: | IV'S/Gtt: |

| Labs: | Notes/Plan: |

Notes/Plan:
- _____
- _____
- _____
- _____
- _____

Nurse Report Sheet

Name:	Code:	Room #:

Allergies:	Isolation:

DX:

PMH:

Neuro:	CV

Resp:	GI/GU:

Skin:	IV'S/Gtt:

Labs:

Notes/Plan:
- _____
- _____
- _____
- _____
- _____

Nurse Report Sheet

Name:

Code:

Room #:

Allergies:

Isolation:

DX:

PMH:

Neuro:

CV

Resp:

GI/GU:

Skin:

IV'S/Gtt:

Labs:

Notes/Plan:

- _____
- _____
- _____
- _____
- _____

Nurse Report Sheet

Name:

Code:

Room #:

Allergies:

Isolation:

DX:

PMH:

Neuro:

CV

Resp:

GI/GU:

Skin:

IV'S/Gtt:

Labs:

Notes/Plan:

- _____
- _____
- _____
- _____
- _____

Nurse Report Sheet

Name:

Code:

Room #:

Allergies:

Isolation:

DX:

PMH:

Neuro:

CV

Resp:

GI/GU:

Skin:

IV'S/Gtt:

Labs:

Notes/Plan:
- _____
- _____
- _____
- _____
- _____

Nurse Report Sheet

Name:

Code:

Room #:

Allergies:

Isolation:

DX:

PMH:

Neuro:

CV

Resp:

GI/GU:

Skin:

IV'S/Gtt:

Labs:

Notes/Plan:

- _____
- _____
- _____
- _____
- _____

Nurse Report Sheet

Name:

Code:

Room #:

Allergies:

Isolation:

DX:

PMH:

Neuro:

CV

Resp:

GI/GU:

Skin:

IV'S/Gtt:

Labs:

Notes/Plan:
- _____
- _____
- _____
- _____
- _____

Nurse Report Sheet

Name:	Code:	Room #:

Allergies:	Isolation:

DX:

PMH:

Neuro:	CV

Resp:	GI/GU:

Skin:	IV'S/Gtt:

Labs:

Notes/Plan:
- _____
- _____
- _____
- _____
- _____

Nurse Report Sheet

Name:

Code:

Room #:

Allergies:

Isolation:

DX:

PMH:

Neuro:

CV

Resp:

GI/GU:

Skin:

IV'S/Gtt:

Labs:

Notes/Plan:

- _____
- _____
- _____
- _____
- _____

Nurse Report Sheet

Name:	Code:	Room #:

Allergies:	Isolation:

DX:

PMH:

Neuro:	CV

Resp:	GI/GU:

Skin:	IV'S/Gtt:

Labs:

Notes/Plan:
- _____
- _____
- _____
- _____
- _____

Nurse Report Sheet

Name:	Code:	Room #:

Allergies:	Isolation:

DX:

PMH:

Neuro:

CV

Resp:

GI/GU:

Skin:

IV'S/Gtt:

Labs:

Notes/Plan:

- _____
- _____
- _____
- _____
- _____

Nurse Report Sheet

Name:

Code:

Room #:

Allergies:

Isolation:

DX:

PMH:

Neuro:

CV

Resp:

GI/GU:

Skin:

IV'S/Gtt:

Labs:

Notes/Plan:

- _____
- _____
- _____
- _____
- _____

Nurse Report Sheet

| Name: | Code: | Room #: |

| Allergies: | Isolation: |

DX:

PMH:

| Neuro: | CV |

| Resp: | GI/GU: |

| Skin: | IV'S/Gtt: |

| Labs: | Notes/Plan:
• _____
• _____
• _____
• _____
• _____ |

Nurse Report Sheet

Name:	Code:	Room #:

Allergies:	Isolation:

DX:

PMH:

Neuro:

CV

Resp:

GI/GU:

Skin:

IV'S/Gtt:

Labs:

Notes/Plan:
- _____
- _____
- _____
- _____
- _____

Nurse Report Sheet

Name:

Code:

Room #:

Allergies:

Isolation:

DX:

PMH:

Neuro:

CV

Resp:

GI/GU:

Skin:

IV'S/Gtt:

Labs:

Notes/Plan:
- _____
- _____
- _____
- _____
- _____

Made in United States
Orlando, FL
18 December 2024